Madison St. Clair's
Get on Up, Let Loose & Dance

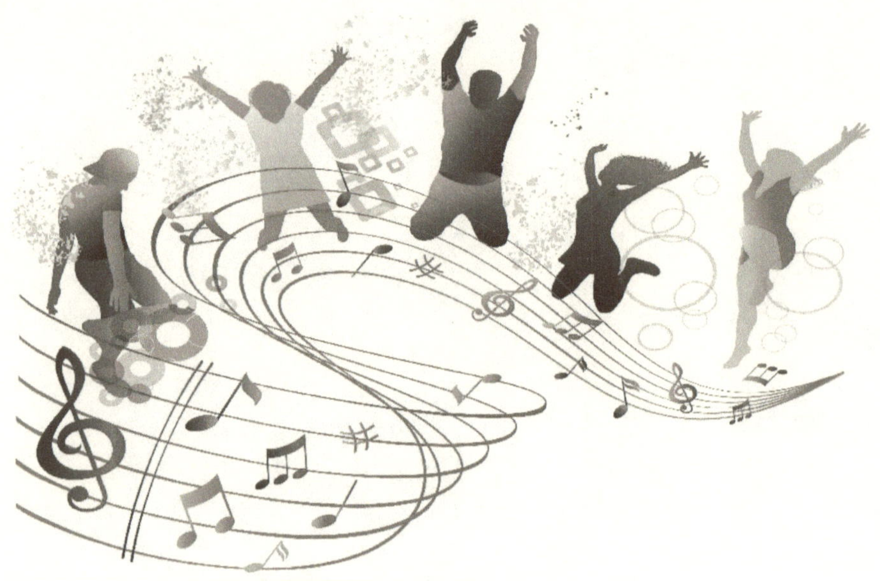

~ Learn to Let Loose ~
3 Simple Tips to Release, Relax &
Rejuvenate

MARGARET P. BEAN

Madison St. Clair's
"Get on Up, Let Loose & Dance"

First Edition
ISBN: 9798641165592

Printed in the United States of America

DEDICATION

I dedicate to my parents my Mother,

the late Evangelist Catherine D. Fulp,

my Father the late Reverend Valdez L. St. Clair.

Thank you, Mr. Walter Nealy Sr., and

my Grandmother the late

Evangelist Margaret G. Williams

I grieve but my grief turns to JOY!

*

To all the families who have had

a family member, friend or

even an acquaintance to succumb to the effects of

Coronavirus (COVID-19)

a worldwide pandemic of 2020.

Be encouraged "for this too shall pass"

Prayers are up for all.

Rest in Peace Ruby Mae Bean &
Frank Mickens

ACKNOWLEDGEMENTS

And I shall say, GOD DID IT
Exceedingly and Abundantly
More than I could have ever imagined
Again….

My life is full of Love

My four lovely Daughters
Ta'Kisha C. Hill, Miecia C. Frost,
Darrell Candance Bean, Danielle C. Bean
My amazing Grand Children
Amajah S. Hill, Semaj S. Hill, Jahlil R. Strayhorn,
Samir L. Frost, Asir C. Abdelaziz, Roman S. Dyer
***

My Brother Tony Nealy & his lovely wife my beautiful
Sister in Love Deborah Nealy nothing but love for you both
***

Thank you for the love and support!
Auntie Barbara & Uncle Robert Jordan,
Auntie Zefrina Taylor, Uncle Wandyful Williams
***

My cousins Wade & Lawanda Isreal,
who always support all I do, legal reviews and always
let me sleep over at the last minute

*Thank you, Cuzzo Timolin Nunn, for the support at every show
rather in NY or MD*

always make time for our breakfast or dinners

means the world to me

*My Franklin Falcons Sharon Hampton Benjamin, Sandra Needy,
Jackie Jacobs & Emma Walker*

appreciate your love and support at every event

*

*My Peeps who always checking on me
Barbara Manley, Jerry White, Karen Sessoms, Barry Alston Ray,
Harmonee Smith, Lisa A. Smith & Pastor Gerald Wayne Smith
Leslie Mauck always got a writer's nugget for me &
Ansonia Saunders, thank you!*

*

My Executive Assistant Julette "GiGi" Mims kept me on point with

the pilot season of Real Talk with Margaret P TV Show

My mentor KaZarr Coleman deeply appreciate you!

*

*Photos Credits
Angela Joy Clemons incredibly talented Boss Lady
Samuel Dickerson
Kevin M Photography*

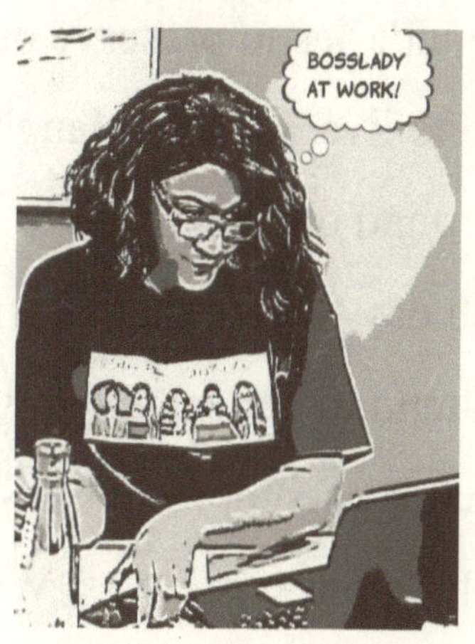

This book was started in 2019 and my life got so busy with a stage play project in New York along with a filming endeavor in Baltimore and the flood gates began to open with several calls leading to major Playwright for hire agreements. I had to step away from this book project. I had overlooked the importance of the result of this project. I personally needed to adhere to the thoughts that would embody this project. I was traveling every weekend and did not realize just how exhausted I was and literally was running on fumes. I am sure you can relate to my zealousness to pursue purpose. My intent in writing this simple 3 step process is to introduce what not only I need to do and have, but so many of you reading this right now. I want you to know the importance of laying down busy and introduce you and I to the 3 R's Rest Relaxation and Rejuvenation. Furthermore, we must stop complaining, learn to relax and set realistic boundaries to preserve our time. We must take time to live, love and laugh. Forgive quickly and surround our selves with positivity and chose each day to give thanks with a grateful heart. Our lives tend to get occupied with "Busy" and we forget that it encompasses "US" smack dead in the middle of our busy lives. We get so busy with work, school, side hustles and grinding for our brands, skills and abilities that we must make time for what is most important, time for family and quality time, planning for free time to relax. I spent some good quality time with my family, to celebrate a birthday but it felt like we were celebrating each other and enjoying some much needed family time, our lives can get so hectic that we don't forget about our family and friends, we just get consumed with what is right in front of us at the moment and forget to prioritize. This day we planned prioritize and didn't allow anything to stop us from all being together "family" we shared great laughter, food, and we Danced and most of all the Love that we shared and the memories we created will forever be cherished. Time is something we cannot get back and it is the most valuable gift we can give. There are somethings that are only a onetime event(s) those onetime experiences we may never get to experience again. Your child's first steps, first birthday and first graduation just to name a few, however; you know your schedule and so learn to adjust accordingly and set priorities. Busy as caused us to lose sight of what is most important. As we misplace importance and quality of life we begin to complain, we forget to relax and our lives are so hectic, we forget that boundaries are necessary to ensure that we take time for ourselves. Our current worldwide situation as adjusted our lives and it's truly sad that life as we knew took an immediate turn that now as lead us to be home bound and under a quarantine since the current events of the Coronavirus (COVID-19) a worldwide pandemic that has taking the world by storm in this year of 2020. Major shutdowns non-essential activities have come to a full halt and by any means necessary *Busy* is now at rest. These events have led to quarantine, curfews and a life threaten virus and deadly occurrences. We are under stay home orders and only essential outside activities for medicines and food. Gas prices are at an all-time low, and airports are empty. You may be wondering how this little book can help. Well glad you asked, while movies, malls and major retailers are closed or have limited access it is definitely a great time to catch up on some reading. Reading a good book is essential right about now and I believe this is a great read for such a time as this to help with taking your mind off the effects of being under a quarantine. It is going to require some activity on your part —a good song, two left feet and a great sense of humor. Music and Dance go hand and hand together they set off a natural inner rhythm. If you take a moment and just listen to your body the greatest instrument ever created, it consists of the heartbeat, which I have six grandchildren and I have had the opportunity to hear their hearts some sounded like running horses, some sounded like thunder and no two roared or rumbled alike. We all have a beat that is a unique rhythm of our own. Fingers snap, Hands clap, Foot stomps and the Mouth when it opens sends a great sound. Go ahead take a moment to just sing and not in the shower right where you are reading this. Yes you! Stop, find your song & sing *(pause for a second)* it was magic wasn't it? Go ahead and smile laugh or even do it again "Sang on! "okay go ahead and admit it, to release an awesome sound it's beautiful or maybe a joyful noise for some. I am in no way saying go out here and quit your day job and become a singer so with that being said you probably should just sing in the car or in the shower, but for this moment "Sang it" but the entire body as a motion that allows you to release all of that inner rhythm. I was feeling a little down and I tuned into a

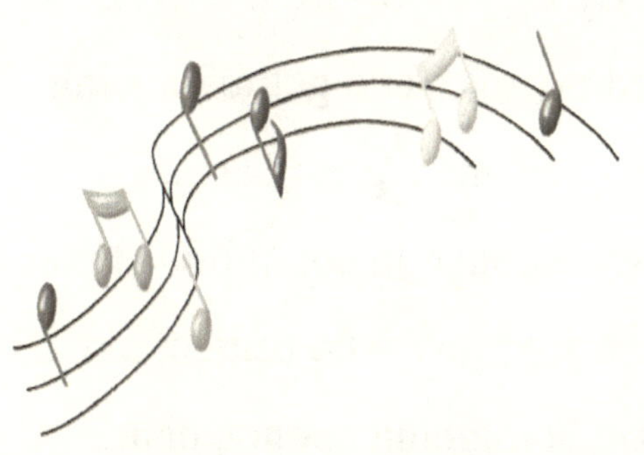

live stream on social media and I am sure he won't mind me giving him credit DJ Vic went live with a musical happy hour to gather family and friends to celebrate a virtual birthday.

The music was great, and all the birthday comments and folks were excited to be connected by a common sound "Music" we all were glad to take a moment to take our minds off the long trying day and celebrate the life of a childhood friend. The music got me not only physically up and moving but my down moment now was a great moment and I was so happy and excited to dance to the sounds of some great music. With the social distancing large events have been postponed and so to keep us connected numerous DJ's and Artist go live on

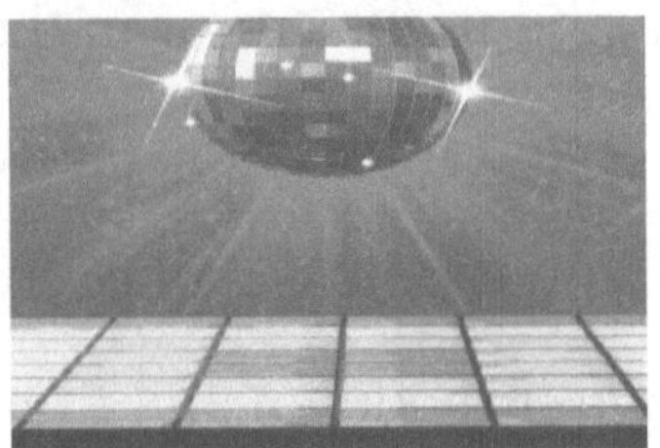

social media with some great music that not only *Got Me Up* and turned my living room into a dance floor, go head try it… I am sure it will do the same for you. I closed my eyes and got to dancing and my down moment became a great Dance moment. One thing we all have in common is two left feet and then there are those who can cut a rug up to a good song. It is something about a dance floor that can allow you to swing sway and fade away to the music. During this uncertain time one thing for sure is that music has been an historical soul soother for centuries. So, I highly recommend that you stop what you are doing and just relax and turn on your favorite song and let the music get you up and dancing. No complaining, no excuses just *Get on Up, Let Loose and Dance* like it is no body's business.

Let us Dance
Margaret P.

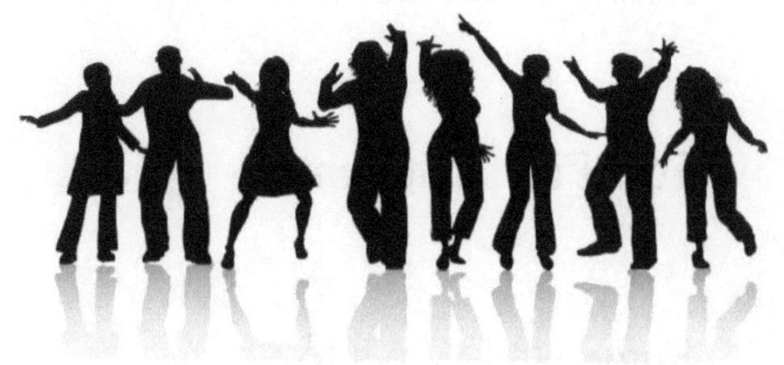

Content

INTRODUCTION

Stop over analyzing everything

Spend less time stressing or worrying about things, you cannot change!

Fall back from the

people in your life who are annoying and constantly complain

Surround yourself with

People

Put the Cell Phone Down and

Read a good book

Realize life is short, so enjoy and

have fun!

Live a life that is authentic to

yourself

Close your eyes Take

control of your thoughts and take

a bubble bath Listen to some music

Learn to Relax

Kick off your shoes

Get on Up, Let Loose & Dance

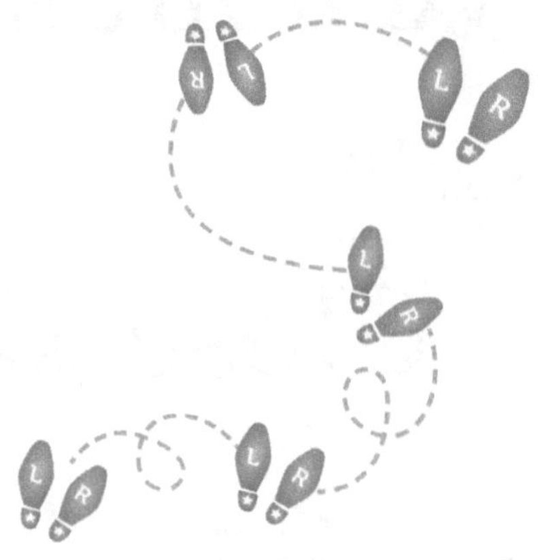

TIP 1

STOP COMPLAINING

Complaining

The expression of dissatisfaction or annoyance about something.

We tend to wake up dreading the day. We must go to work or school and when we walk out the door, the first thought is to complain about having to get up, having to go to work, or just having to start the day. Instead of always complaining "Stop" "Look Around" and "Enjoy" the fact that you are up! Open the blinds let the sunshine in and enjoy the warmth of the sun on your face. Walk in the bathroom look in the mirror and say Good morning self! In addition, let us start this day off right, you choose your attitude for today.

<u>It is okay to Choose</u>

- Today I choose to be Happy

- I choose not to Stress

- I choose to live life on Purpose

- I choose not to complain about the things that I cannot control.

- Stress and Complaining will not rule my day

- Today is going to be a Great Day!

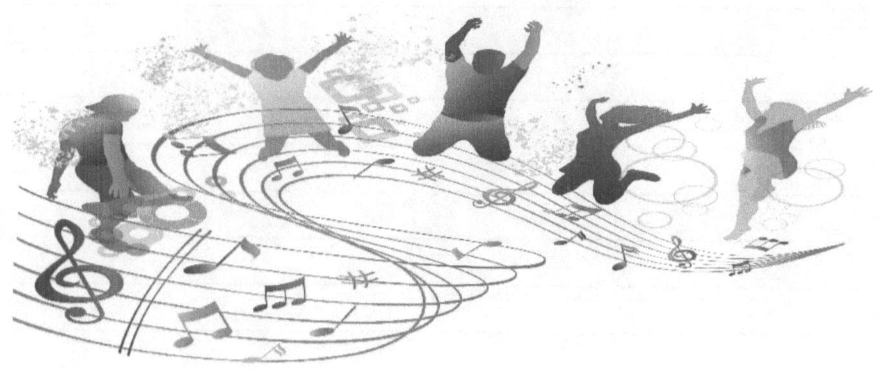

Write down some good thoughts and ponder on those for a while. Choose things that make you smile versus complaining!

TIP 2

Learn to Relax

RELAX

Make or become less tense or anxious.

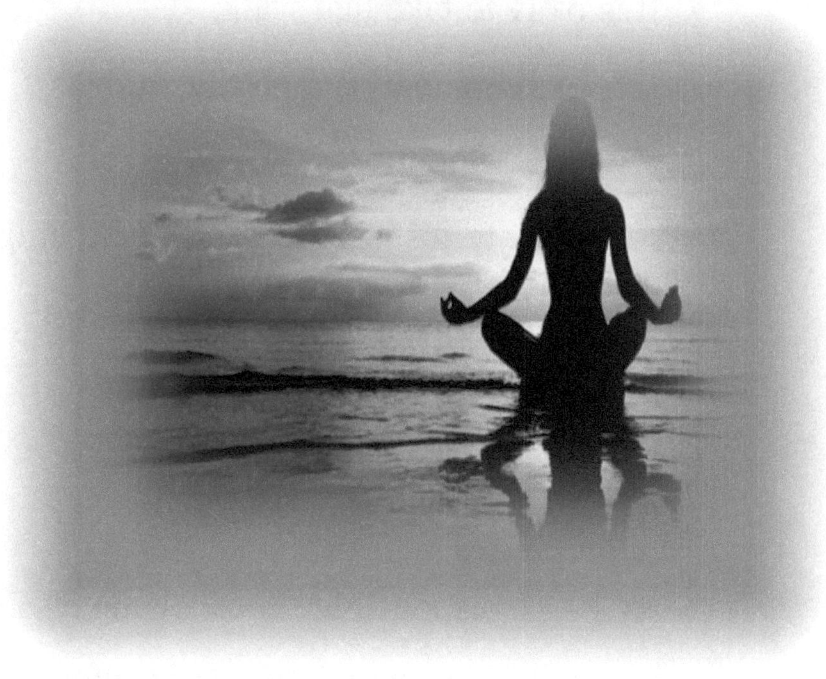

Learn to Relax!

Be anxious for nothing – Once again, "You" have a choice in the matter – Choose to lighten up and Relax.

- It is okay to take that walk,
- It is okay to be in DO Not Disturb mode… - Phone Off!
- It is okay to just sit back and do nothing
- Enjoy your deck or patio in that lawn chair you never use
- It is okay to say NO!

You are **<u>NOT</u>** responsible for everyone else's responsibilities, happiness, or journey

<u>Key Point:</u> There is only so much you can do in one day!

Stop!

Drop and "Take a Nap" if you need to

Be sure that you are well rested and not
feeling anxious about anything take a hot bath
and just relax and enjoy the sound of the
water and lay in the bubbles – it is okay to
take time for you!
Learn how to loosen up from
the tensions that can fill the day.

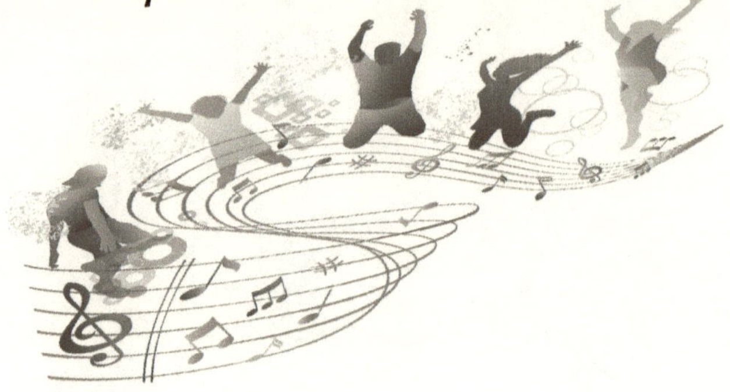

Make a list of what you like to do to Relax

❖ _______________________________________

❖ _______________________________________

❖ _______________________________________

❖ _______________________________________

❖ _______________________________________

❖ _______________________________________

TIP 3

Learn to
Set Boundaries

Creating and Setting

Healthy Boundaries for your life

"Is OKAY"

Stop trying to please people and

Begin to live life on your own terms

[Validation is for Parking]

It is Okay to make time for you first

It is Okay for you to say NO

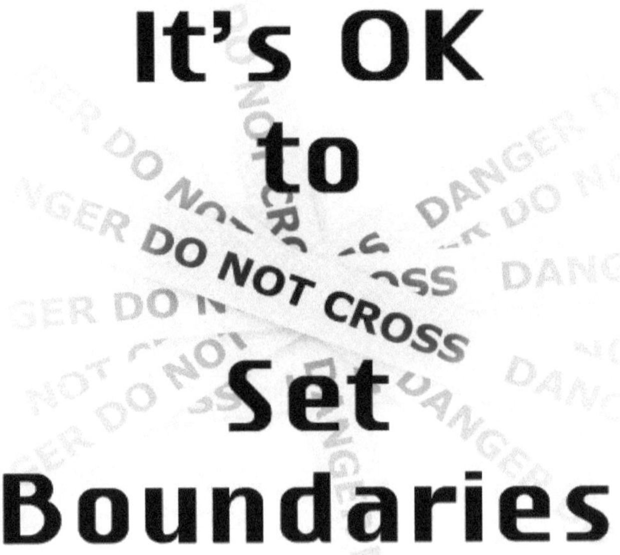

- It is Okay to put you first.

- Protect your time – do not overcommit.

- Ask for space – we all need our own time.

- Know your limits.

- Stay firm in your conviction.

- Understand that your needs are important.

- Seek to take care of yourself.

- Set Priorities.

- Communicate and express your feelings.

- Keep the Balance of work, home & free time.

- Give yourself permission to do what is best for you!

Separating who we are

what we feel or think, from the feelings and

thoughts of others

Respect my Space

Allow yourself to process

It is Okay to Say No!

Avoid Negative Environments

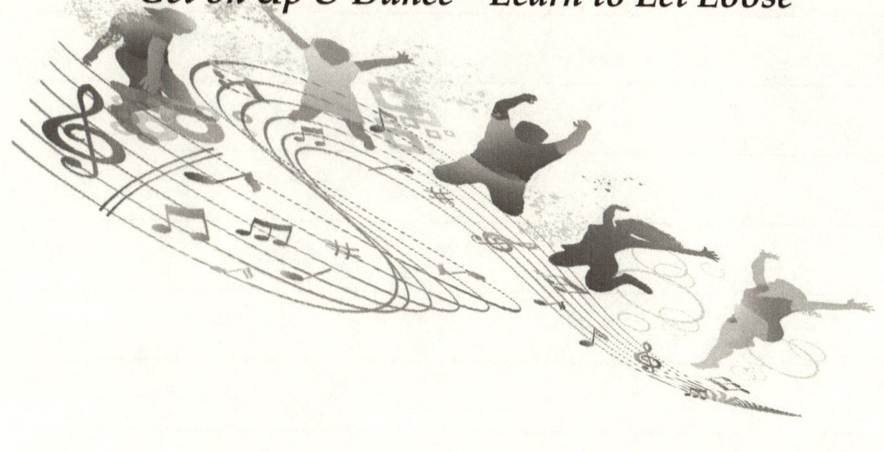

Set Boundaries that Protect your

Space

Time

Peace &

Priorities

Few final thoughts …..This is a short read interactive book and so my intent was to provide some very basic steps and I did not wont to overload you with a heavy content read, just something light and easy to have fun with however; I hope that something you read inspires you to take a moment each day and to choose your course. Do not allow your 24 hours to get or be consumed with busy, stuff, worry, anxiety or things that steal your joy, your smile and positive energy, limit your calendar appointments and matter a fact schedule an appointment for you and take some time to enjoy this life. I am grateful for this opportunity to speak a word of encouragement into your lives. My goal is always to encourage, inspire, build, and strengthen others with positive words, vibes, and actions.

During this time of uncertainty of events there is one thing that is certain that our creator, as not to offend anyone's beliefs I personally call him "God" while some may call him Allah, Jehovah or your higher power – tap into that spiritual place and seek peace, wisdom, joy, and all things needed to carry out this life journey.

Things certainly have changed in all our lives and so stay focused, relax, release, and rejuvenate by any means necessary please be careful, mask up and reenter society with caution. We will have a new norm which none of us know what that may look like; however, do not get so "Busy" that you forget to take a moment to Get on Up, Let Loose and Dance!

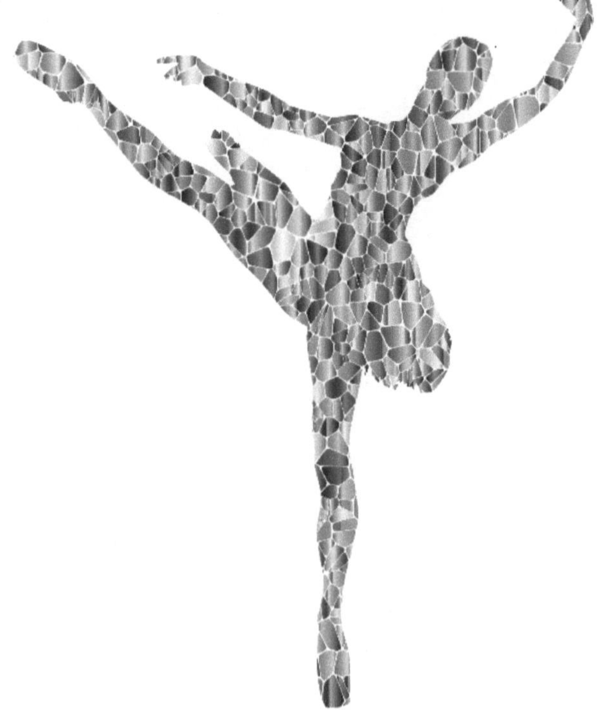

1. Hot bubble bath or shower
   with aromatherapy candles
2. Take a long walk or ride a bike
3. Exercise and Dance
4. Reduce stress
5. Speak positive
6. Read a good book
7. Make a list of things you want to do and
   then just do them
8. Pamper yourself (facial, spa day, pedicure)
9. Take a mental health day to just do nothing
10. Spend quality time with loved one's

In conclusion I admonish you to loosen up and take time to write out your thoughts on the work sheets and just take moments to "Dance" if you like post positive confessions in your bathroom mirror so when you wake up and start your day it's with positive affirmation for a good day, speak to your day "I Choose a Great day!"…. It is okay to repeat positivity daily and it is Okay to Stop Complaining, learn how to Relax and finally it is necessary to set Boundaries it is alright to protect your space and peace.

 God chooses the Ordinary to do the Extraordinary for His own purposes and in that He gives you a gift and a calling that is irrevocable. So, even with life gives you difficulties and change, the call of God is the one consistent thing.

Margaret P. Bean, Multi Published Author brings her Soul-Satisfying brand to the content she creates. Her soul stirring traditional published "Seeking God's Wisdom" was followed up by two other phenomenal self-published titles "Raising the Standard in your Walk with the Lord" and the diverse writings of "Madison St. Clair's Turning Points, Short Stories, Poems & Silent moments"

In 2017 Margaret's endeavours took her into Playwrighting & Directing her first stage play titled "The Game Changer" which ran for two years and toured MD, NY, DC and back to NY.

Margaret is currently working on a play project titled "Sister Code There's Rules to this thing" there are other projects underway so be sure to visit my website for updates and new releases.

Margaret is an energetic and gifted speaker. Her message of "Self-Discovery Through Life's Adversities" is quickly gaining traction among an array of audiences. Margaret is available to speak to organizations, churches, clubs, educational institutions, and all receptive audiences.

Margaret is pursuing her passion "MPB Entertainment" with the intent of creating quality content for not only the stage, but with great hopes of the big screen and television next.

Stay in Contact with Margaret by visiting the website: www.msmargaretpbean.com, email for bookings or speaking engagements at madisun516@gmail.com, follow her on Instagram, Twitter and look her up on Facebook.

I want to personally take this time to say that I sincerely appreciate the support of my family, few friends & faithful supporters, of my endeavours your time and willingness to support rather reading my published works or attending a show means the world to me. My heart smiles and I am incredibly grateful for your

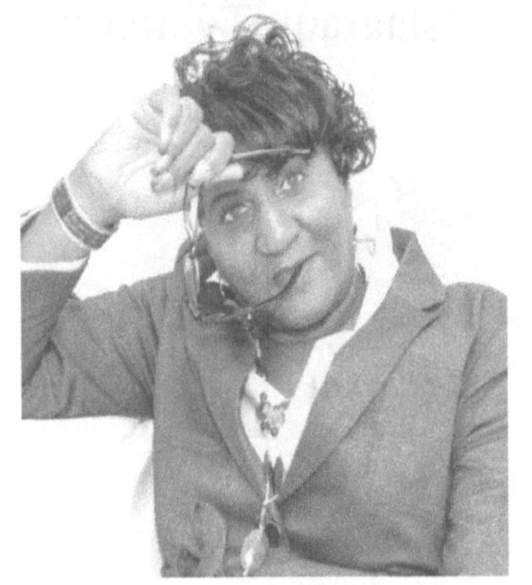

continued support and I look forward to providing you with greater original creative content.

Much Love, Margaret P. Bean

A Woman About Her Business!